Essential Skills Series

Essential Skills Book 7

Twenty-five Passages
with Questions for
Developing the Six
Essential Categories
of Comprehension

Walter Pauk, Ph.D.
Director, Reading-
Study Center
Cornell University

Jamestown Publishers

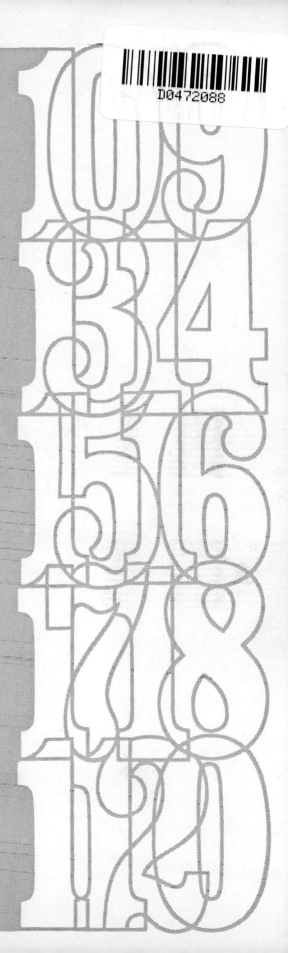

PREFACE

Why do boys shoot baskets over and over again and girls skate and reskate the same routine? These beginners know that practice makes perfect. Not only do beginners know this, but pros do too. For what other reason do they work at baseball and football week after week before the opening dates?

The pros know the value of practice, but they also know the value of something else. They know that practice without *instruction* and *guidance* does not automatically lead to improvement. That's why they have the best coaches that money can buy.

And so it is with developing the skills of reading. There must be the right kind of practicing and the right kind of coaching.

First, a word about practice. In this book the right kind of practice is provided by 25 articles, highly interesting and carefully selected. Here is material enough on which to grow and keep growing.

Now about coaching! Good coaching takes the form of instruction and guidance. In this book the instruction is straightforward and uncomplicated. It puts you directly on the right track, and better still, you are kept on the right track by two unusual systems of guidance. The first system is the uniquely-designed, six-way-question format which makes sure that every ounce of practice is directed toward improvement. Nothing is wasted!

The second system of guidance is the Diagnostic Chart. This chart is no ordinary gimmick. In truth, it provides the most dignified form of diagnosis and guidance yet devised. It provides instantaneous and continuous diagnosis and gentle but certain self-guidance. It yields information directly to the student. There is no middleman. No one needs to needle him. This form of self-guidance leads to the goal of all education: the goal of self-learning.

Now, I want to make some acknowledgements, especially to the students who were the guinea pigs. Afterwards I told them so, but they said, "We didn't mind even then. And now that it is over, we're all the happier because we know how much we've learned." But what the students did not know was how much I learned from them. For this I thank them all, class after class.

I direct especial thanks to Linda Browning for handling the almost countless number of selections, writing and refining the questions and making sure that the series kept moving: all, a most demanding task.

Finally, I am most grateful to authors, editors and publishers who have generously given permission to quote and reprint in this book from works written and published by them. The books quoted in the text and used as sources of reading extracts are listed in the back of the booklet. — W.P.

Essential Skills Series
ES-7, Book 7, Grade 6A, ISBN 0-89061-106-8

CONTENTS

ORGANIZATION OF THE BOOKLETS

Selection Criteria. Twenty-five of the very best articles obtainable were selected for each booklet. Each article had to meet, at least, the following criteria: *high interest level, appropriate readability level,* and *factual accuracy of contents.*

High interest was assured by choosing passages from popular magazines that appeal to a wide range of readers. The readability level of each passage was determined by the use of the Dale-Chall readability formula, thus enabling the arrangement of passages on a single grade level within each booklet. The factual accuracy of the passages is high because they were written by professional writers whose works are recognized and respected.

The Questions. At the end of each passage there are six questions to answer. The six questions will always be within the framework of the following six categories: subject matter; main ideas; supporting details; conclusions; clarifying devices; and vocabulary in context. By repeated practice with questions within these six essential categories, students will develop an active, searching attitude when reading other expository prose. These questions will help them become aware of what they are reading at the time of the actual perception of the words and phrases, thus building high comprehension.

The Diagnostic Chart. Fast and sure improvement in reading comprehension can be made by using the Diagnostic Chart to identify relative strengths and weaknesses. The Diagnostic Chart is a very efficient instrument. Here is how it works.

The questions for every passage are always in the same order. For example, the question designed to teach the skill of recognizing the *main idea* is always in the number two position, and the skill of drawing *conclusions* is always in the number four position, and so on.

The Diagnostic Chart functions automatically when the letters of answers are placed in the proper spaces. Even after completing one passage, the chart will reveal the types of questions answered correctly, as well as the types answered incorrectly. But more important for the long run is that the chart will identify the types of questions that are missed consistently. Once a weakness (in drawing conclusions, for example) is ascertained, the following procedure is recommended: First, the student should reread the question; then, with the correct answer in mind, he should reread the entire passage trying to perceive how the author actually did lead to or imply the correct conclusion. Second, on succeeding passages, he should put forth extra effort to answer correctly the questions pertaining to drawing conclusions. Third, if the difficulty continues, he should arrange a conference with his teacher.

TEACHING THE SIX ESSENTIAL SKILLS

What reading skills does a person have to know to gain meaning from factual prose? To gain meaning, most people would have to know, at least, six essential skills. They would have to know how to concentrate to glean the subject matter, to grasp main ideas, to relate supporting details to main ideas and sub-ideas, to draw conclusions, to recognize clarifying devices, and to unlock the meaning of words. Let's take a closer look at these skills.

Concentration/Subject Matter

There is no problem that I hear more frequently than, "I can't concentrate!" Fortunately, there's a sure, fast cure. There is no better magic for gaining concentration while reading than this one: After reading the first few lines of a selection, softly ask yourself this question, "What is this article about?" In other words, "What's the general subject matter?"

If you don't ask this question, here's what will generally happen: Your eyes will move across the lines of print while your mind is still entertaining the lingering thoughts of a previous conversation or daydream.

If you ask the question, however, you will almost always arrive at an answer, thus capturing concentration. Let's see whether or not this technique works. Here are the first lines of an article:

> Wood ducks are the most beautiful ducks in America. Once they
> were rare. Now — if you have sharp eyes and can keep quiet — you
> might see them in almost any woodland, along streams and ponds.

Obviously, you can say with a great degree of assurance that the author is going to talk about the wood duck. Now that your mind is on the trail, the chances are great it will follow the author's ideas paragraph after paragraph, thereby *concentrating* on the development of the subject matter.

Let's try the technique again. Here are a few lines from another article:

> Of all the little animals in the world, the Columbian ground squirrel
> is one of the liveliest and friendliest. He is nicknamed "picket pin"
> because he sits as stiff and straight as a stake on the ground.

Again, you probably experienced no trouble at all zeroing in on the subject matter: the Columbian ground squirrel.

The Main Idea

Once the general subject matter has been quickly ascertained, it is easier for the mind to grapple with the next question: What is the author's main idea? What point is he trying to get across?

With such questions in mind, it is surprising how often an answer pops up. When no questions are asked, it seems that everything is on the same level — nothing stands out.

Let us peruse another short excerpt, this time for the main idea.

> Wood ducks never nest on the ground as most ducks do, but in a
> big hole in a tree. Trees with big holes in them are hard to find.

Since you don't have the full article to read, may I make this comment: The main point that the author is making is that with the scarcity of old, dead trees with holes in them, we will have fewer and fewer wood ducks.

Thus, we see that by asking questions, reading becomes a two-way street. When we talk with the author, the article seems to come to life. Reading then becomes an exciting and enjoyable experience.

Supporting Details

Are we interested in details? Of course we are! In longer articles, main ideas and sub-ideas are the bones, the skeleton of the articles. The details are the flesh which gives articles completeness, fullness and life.

Details are used almost entirely to support the main idea and sub-ideas. Consequently, the term *supporting details* is appropriate. These supporting details come in various forms, but the most common forms are: examples, definitions, comparisons and contrasts, repetitions and descriptions.

The author of "The Wood Duck" has supplied us with enough information so that we know the article is about wood ducks. Next, he made sure that we understood the point that without "trees with big holes in them" the wood duck will not nest; thus, there would be fewer wood ducks.

Having gotten us interested in this unique problem, he then supplied details on how we could provide "trees with big holes in them." He *described* how we could build a wood duck nesting box. Here's the excerpt:

> Why don't you and your parents put up wood duck nesting boxes
> right now? It would be about 2 feet high and 10 inches square. Make
> the entry hole about four inches in diameter. Use rough lumber on the
> inside so the ducklings can climb up the sides to the hole. Put wood
> shavings in the bottom in which the duck will lay her eggs. To keep her
> eggs warm, she covers them with her own feathers. If you don't have a
> tree near the water, you'll need a post. Place the box 10 to 30 feet high.

You can see in the above example how important details are in telling a story. Details enable the reader to visualize what's going on, how to do something, how to take action, and so forth.

In any article of length, there will be some or many sub-ideas. It is important to be sufficiently wary so as not to mistake a sub-idea for a main idea. One way to distinguish between the two is as follows: The main idea pertains to the entire article, whereas the sub-idea pertains only to a portion of it. Notice that in the following example the sub-idea is about the food which wood ducks eat. The entire article is *not* about food, so it is *not* the main idea. In most cases you will see that a sub-idea takes the space of one paragraph.

The main purpose for including the following excerpts is to show how the author clusters and organizes his supporting details around the relatively minor sub-ideas which are stated in topic sentences. In other words, a sub-idea is the nucleus which holds a body of details together.

> Wood ducks like to eat acorns and all kinds of nuts. Their stomachs (or gizzards) have such powerful muscles that they can break the hardest nuts, some that you could barely crack with a hammer! Wood ducks like berries, duckweed and insects. But best of all they like to eat spiders — that's ice cream to them.

The author, after adding to the article a brief but detailed description of some food which wood ducks eat, continues on to describe how the newly hatched ducklings get down to the ground from some dizzy heights. Here are more details clustered around another sub-idea.

> Sometimes they nest in holes up in trees that are twice as high as a flagpole. Just think, the baby ducklings must jump to the ground the day they hatch. Usually they don't get hurt, though, because they're light, like little puffs of cotton. The mother stands at the foot of the tree and calls and calls. Like little paratroopers, the ducklings peek out of the hole, then jump quickly, one right after the other, to join their mother, who must hurry them to the pond where they're safe.

Thus, one of the main functions of *supporting details* is to give some dimension to an article. Otherwise, it would be a rather uninteresting, skimpy statement of one main idea together with its bare-boned sub-ideas. The examples, descriptions, explanations, etc., are what give life to the article.

Conclusions

As a reader moves through an article, understanding the main idea, the sub-ideas and their supporting details, it is only natural for him to anticipate a conclusion to the author's story. Such anticipation is part of the sport of reading. Frequently, though, the author provides the reader with a conclusion. In such an event, the joy of reading lies in the fact that the reader was able to anticipate accurately the conclusion. In the event that a conclusion is not stated, the perceptive reader will be able to seize the implied conclusion.

From the excerpts just read about the wood duck, the conclusion is in the form of having the reader visualize the pleasure of having a wood duck to observe. The concluding sentence is this:

> If you're lucky, though, and if your (duck) house is in place before the ice melts, you will have a wood duck family in the summer.

In another selection entitled "From Pond to Prairie," the author has this as his conclusion:

> Finally, there is no longer much open water. The pond has disappeared. Depending on the kinds of plants that have filled it, the pond

> may be called a bog or a marsh. As changes continue for many more
> years, the bog may become a forest.

The reader who reads with speed and comprehension is the reader who, like a detective, follows the maze of ideas and details and descriptions, but who is always thinking, "Where is the author leading me? What's his final point? What's his conclusion?" And, of course, like a detective, the reader must continually anticipate a conclusion, always correcting or reinforcing his anticipations as he takes in more and more of the story or selection.

Clarifying Devices

Just as the name implies, the author uses everything that he can possibly think of to make his points clear and interesting. In a sense, the much-mentioned *topic sentence* may be thought of as a clarifying device. By placing it at the very beginning of a passage, the author provides the reader with an immediate point of focus, as well as a definite statement from which the reader can anticipate what is to come.

But usually, by clarifying devices, we mean the author's use of literary devices, such as transitional words and phrases which keep the ideas, sub-ideas and details in proper relationship.

To make ideas as well as details clear and interesting in themselves, authors frequently use additional literary devices such as the *metaphor*, an example of which follows: But best of all they like to eat spiders — *that's ice cream to them.*

Another literary device which authors frequently use is the *simile: Like little paratroopers,* the ducklings peek out of the hole, then jump quickly, one right after the other. The simile about the paratroopers provides the reader with familiar material which helps him to visualize the scene more graphically and vividly.

In addition to transitional words and phrases, metaphors and similes, there are many other types of *clarifying devices*. Another cluster of clarifying devices are the organizational patterns. One such pattern is the chronological pattern in which the events unfold in the order of time; that is, one thing happens first, and then another, and another, and so forth.

The time pattern may give structure and control to an incident that takes place in a span of five minutes or to an historical era which may span hundreds of years. Or, used in another way, the time pattern may be the vehicle used to sequence the activities of an animal from birth to death or even to delineate the sequence of events in a transition.

By knowing some of these clarifying devices, you will be able to recognize them in the selections that you read, and, by recognizing them, you will be able to read with greater comprehension and with greater speed.

Vocabulary in Context

Of course, if a reader doesn't understand some of the words and terms in a selection, he runs the risk of misconstruing the author's ideas. It should be obvious that a reader should pause to look up in a dictionary the words and terms that he does not know.

However, what is not so obvious is that many readers who may understand the general meaning of a word don't stop to look up such a word to ascertain its *precise* meaning.

When such a reader imposes upon a generally understood word his rather general understanding, he may end up with a blurred picture of the idea. Whereas, when he imposes a precise and full meaning upon a word, his chances of emerging with a precise and full picture of the author's idea are immensely enhanced.

For example, in the following excerpt are two common words which most people feel they already know. Consequently, they don't see any reason for any dictionary work. Nevertheless, few people know them with the precision the words deserve.

> Depending on the kinds of plants that have filled it, the pond may be called a *bog* or a *marsh*.

Do you know the difference between a bog and a marsh? Is there a difference? If so, what is it? Would your mental picture be different if you knew?

Looking up words which you think you already know might be far more rewarding than simply seeking to add more totally unknown words to your vocabulary. In other words, strive for a smaller but *precise* vocabulary, rather than for a broader but slightly blurred vocabulary.

Looking up words you feel you already know will probably take more discipline than looking up unknown words. Here are some words that are likely to be unknown; so, turning to the dictionary is almost a reflex action:

> Nothing could appear more *benign* than a field aglow with daisies, goldenrod and Queen Anne's lace.

> *Sphinxlike*, it crouches among the flowers until the desired insect wanders within reach.

Thus, the dictionary is the stock market where we can exchange fuzzy meanings and soft meanings for precise meanings and where we can acquire new meanings for unknown words and all this at no cost other than a flip of the finger.

GETTING THE MOST OUT OF THIS BOOKLET

The steps given below for you to follow could be called "tricks of the trade." Your teachers might call them "rules for learning." It doesn't matter what they are called. What does matter is that they work.

Think About the Title

A good reader we know told us about a "trick" he uses every time he reads. He said, "The first thing I do is read the title. Then I spend a few moments thinking about it."

Writers spend a lot of time thinking up good titles. They try to pack as much meaning as possible into them. It makes sense, then, for the reader to spend a few seconds trying to get the full meaning out. These few moments of thought give the reader a head start on the story.

Thinking about the title can help you in another way, too. It starts you off concentrating on the story before you actually begin reading it. Why does this happen? Thinking about the title fills your head so full of thoughts about the story that there's no room for anything else to get in to break concentration.

If you have trouble concentrating when you read, try this step. It works!

The Dot System

Here is a step that will speed up your reading and build comprehension at the same time.

After spending a few moments with the title, read *quickly* through the passage. Then, without looking back, answer the six questions, using a dot. For each question, place a dot in the box beside the answer of your choice. The dots will be your "unofficial" answers.

The dot system helps by making you work a little harder on your first, *fast* reading. The effort you make to grasp and retain ideas makes you a better reader.

The Check-Mark System

After you have answered all of the questions with a dot, read the story again, *carefully*. This time, make your final answers to the questions using a check mark (✓). For each question, place a check mark in the box next to the answer of your choice. The answers with the check marks are the ones that will count toward your score.

The Diagnostic Chart

Now, transfer your final answers to the diagnostic chart on page 64. Use the column of boxes under number 1 for the answers to the first passage; use the column of boxes under number 2 for the answers to the second story, and so on.

Write the letter of your answer in the *upper* portion of each block.

Correct your answers using the answer key on page 63. When scoring your answers, do *not* use an x for *incorrect* or a c for *correct*. Instead, follow this method. If your answer is correct, make no mark in the answer block; leave it alone. If your answer is *in*correct, write the letter of the correct answer in the *lower* portion of the block, underneath your wrong answer.

Properly used, then, the answer column for each story will show not only your incorrect answers, but also what the correct answers should be. This sets the stage for the next step.

Taking Corrective Action

Your incorrect answers give you a real opportunity for self-learning. Take this opportunity to study your wrong answers. Go back to the original question and read the correct answer several times. With the correct answer in mind, go back to the story itself. Read to see why the approved answer is best. Try to see where you made your mistake. Try to see why you chose a wrong answer.

Graphing Your Progress

Underneath the diagnostic chart on page 64 is a progress graph for you to use. For each story, put an *x* where the lines cross to show your score. Join the *x*'s as you go; plot a line showing your progress.

The Steps in a Nutshell

Here's a quick review of the steps you have just read:

1. **Think About the Title.** Get from the title all the meaning the writer put into it.

2. **The Dot System.** After your first, fast reading, answer the six questions using a dot. The dots are your unofficial answers.

3. **The Check-Mark System.** Read the passage again, carefully this time. Put a check mark (✓) in the box beside your final answer.

4. **The Diagnostic Chart.** Record your final answers in the upper blocks on the chart on page 64. Use the column of blocks under the number of the passage you have just read.

5. **The Answer Key.** Using the key on page 63, correct your answers. Leave correct answers alone. Write the approved answers in the boxes underneath your incorrect ones.

6. **Taking Correct Action.** Study all of your wrong answers. Read the story again. Try to see why and where you were wrong.

7. **Graphing Your Progress.** Plot your scores on the graph on page 64. Join the *x*'s to show your line of progress.

1. THE GIANT GRAY WHALE

Each year in the autumn, hundreds of people from miles around go to San Diego, California, to see one of the strangest parades in the world. The marchers are not soldiers, clowns or four-legged animals as you might expect. They are giant California gray whales. The whales are on the last lap of a long, long journey that takes them almost 8,000 miles.

One by one, two by two, or in groups, the 45-foot-long whales swim through the water close to the California coast. They are returning from their summer feeding grounds in the far North. All summer they have been living in the ice-cold Arctic Ocean and Bering Sea close to the shores of Siberia. Then they head for their winter homes in the shallow lagoons of Mexico's Baja California and stay there until spring.

The gray whale gets its name from the thousands of barnacles that cling to its body. The barnacles form a kind of crust giving the whales a grayish color.

Whales are mammals so they have lungs and must breathe air. The spectators who come to see the whales' migration like to watch the whales come to the surface for air about every fifteen minutes. But before a whale takes in fresh air, it blows out the stale air from its lungs through two blowholes on the top of its head. This is why the whalers of old cried "Thar she blows!" when they spotted the great twin plumes of mist bursting from the sea.

1. Choose the best title.
   ☐ a. What To Do with Whale Oil
   ☐ b. The Gray Travelers
   ☐ c. The Dying Out of the Gray Whale
   ☐ d. Population Explosion — The Gray Whale

2. Every fall and spring the gray whale
   ☐ a. can be easily hunted.
   ☐ b. goes into hibernation.
   ☐ c. mates.
   ☐ d. migrates to new waters.

3. The gray whale gets its color from
   ☐ a. the barnacles on its body.
   ☐ b. the fish it eats.
   ☐ c. living in cold water.
   ☐ d. seaweed growing on its body.

4. In the spring the gray whales
   ☐ a. migrate to Antarctica.
   ☐ b. return to the Arctic Ocean.
   ☐ c. hunt for porpoise.
   ☐ d. bear their young.

5. In the last paragraph, the writer is telling us how whales
   ☐ a. swim.
   ☐ b. eat their food.
   ☐ c. keep their bodies warm.
   ☐ d. breathe.

6. A shallow lagoon is not very
   ☐ a. cold.
   ☐ b. deep.
   ☐ c. salty.
   ☐ d. warm.

CATEGORIES OF COMPREHENSION QUESTIONS

No. 1: Subject Matter   No. 3: Supporting Details   No. 5: Clarifying Devices
No. 2: Main Idea   No. 4: Conclusion   No. 6: Vocabulary in Context

---

2. A 3,000-POUND TONGUE!

The gray whale does not have teeth. Instead, it has hundreds of long, flexible, bonelike plates or strips hanging from its upper jaw. These plates are called baleen (buh LEEN).

When the whale feeds, it scoops in huge loads of small shrimp, clams, crabs and eel grass from the ocean floor. A great amount of water and sand are also scooped up along with this food. The food particles must then be filtered, or screened, and held in the mouth by the baleen. The water and sand that have been filtered are pushed out of the whale's mouth by its huge tongue. The tongue then licks the food off the baleen. (Some whales' tongues may weigh 3,000 pounds!)

Often the whale will "stand" on its tail. This probably helps the animal shake the large amount of food into its stomach.

The whale is very well adapted to its life in the ocean. Pumping its powerful tail in an up-and-down motion, it moves along at about 4 knots. That's about 4-1/2 miles an hour. But if the whale has to, it can speed through the water at 10 knots for periods of up to an hour. Some gray whales have even been known to reach speeds of 30 knots when breaching into the air.

Some scientists believe the leaping helps a whale to navigate by giving it a look at the waters around it. Underwater, however, the whale finds its way by using its sensitive sonar system. First, the whale makes a series of clicking noises. These sounds travel through the water and bounce off objects in the area. By listening for the echo, the whale can tell if anything is in front of it and can then avoid swimming into it. Without this sonar, whales would never be able to make their long migrations.

1. This passage is about the gray whale and
   □ a. how it mates.
   □ b. its life in the ocean.
   □ c. where it is mostly found.
   □ d. the scientist that discovered it.

2. According to this story, the gray whale is well adapted for
   □ a. life in the ocean.
   □ b. deep sea diving.
   □ c. life in cold waters.
   □ d. feeding its young.

3. The strips hanging from the whale's upper jaw are called
   □ a. teeth.
   □ b. baleen.
   □ c. sonar.
   □ d. standings.

4. The writer suggests that sonar is used when the whale
   □ a. mates.
   □ b. eats.
   □ c. travels.
   □ d. sleeps.

5. Some whales reach thirty knots when "breaching into the air." This means the whale is
   □ a. swimming along the surface.
   □ b. floating on its back.
   □ c. falling from the air to the water.
   □ d. leaping from the water into the air.

6. Another word for filtered found within the same sentence is
   □ a. food.   □ c. screened.
   □ b. particles.   □ d. baleen.

CATEGORIES OF COMPREHENSION QUESTIONS

No. 1: Subject Matter   No. 3: Supporting Details   No. 5: Clarifying Devices
No. 2: Main Idea   No. 4: Conclusion   No. 6: Vocabulary in Context

3. WHALES NEED PROTECTION

When a female whale (cow) is ready to give birth, she may head for the open sea or she may choose a far-off corner in one of the Baja California lagoons. Usually, though, the cow will choose to give birth in the lagoon entrance. After a cow mates and is fertilized, a year will pass before she gives birth to her calf. Since a female whale has only one calf at a time, the number of gray whales does not increase quickly.

Hunters, over a period of years, have killed too many of these slow-breeding whales. In the late 1930s, the International Whaling Commission declared the gray whale nearly extinct and voted to protect it from all hunters. This meant that people could not kill gray whales at any time or anywhere.

Mexico has given some help to the gray whale. It has provided a safe lagoon for mating and calving and does not permit hunting. The gray whales have been able to make a comeback. There are anywhere from 6,000 to 18,000 of them alive today. The threat of extinction is gone — for now.

In the United States, a whale bill was introduced to Congress. This bill seeks to protect all whales for at least ten years. Although the gray whale is temporarily safe, many other species are endangered and need our help to survive. There are several ways that this can be done. Experts have pointed out that the dozens of products made from whale oil, such as candles, varnish, lipsticks and linoleum, could easily be manufactured from other substances. The pet-food industry could find substitutes for whale meat. If other materials were used for these products, the killing of whales could be decreased.

In 1966 the Soviet Union banned the catching and killing of the dolphin. Couldn't they, and we, do the same for endangered whales?

1. This passage discusses the
   ☐ a. blue whale.
   ☐ b. killer whale.
   ☐ c. great white whale.
   ☐ d. gray whale.

2. Whales are becoming extinct because of
   ☐ a. years of hunting.
   ☐ b. disease.
   ☐ c. lack of food.
   ☐ d. polluted water.

3. A female whale is called a
   ☐ a. mare.
   ☐ b. cow.
   ☐ c. bull.
   ☐ d. calf.

4. The next to last paragraph suggests that whales are used in the manufacture of
   ☐ a. cloth.   ☐ c. pet food.
   ☐ b. gum.   ☐ d. candy.

5. The gray whales are making a comeback which means that
   ☐ a. they will attack anything.
   ☐ b. the whales are good swimmers.
   ☐ c. they will soon be extinct.
   ☐ d. they are increasing in number.

6. In this article calving means
   ☐ a. giving birth.
   ☐ b. growing.
   ☐ c. killing.
   ☐ d. hunting.

CATEGORIES OF COMPREHENSION QUESTIONS

No. 1: Subject Matter   No. 3: Supporting Details   No. 5: Clarifying Devices
No. 2: Main Idea   No. 4: Conclusion   No. 6: Vocabulary in Context

4. THE FIGHTING BASS

Every day, for all the animals below the still waters of a peaceful lake, there is a life and death struggle going on. Each animal, whether big or small, is living its own life cycle. An animal is born, develops movement, learns to catch food, mates and sometimes dies naturally of old age.

More often, however, he becomes food for another animal. Thus, not all the animals complete their life cycles because animal life is interdependent. That is, life lives off other life. Sometimes an animal is the hunter and at other times, the prey.

The largemouth bass is found in many freshwater lakes in this country. Whether in dark depths or sunny shallow water, weedy swamp or upland stream, the largemouth bass — inch for inch, pound for pound — is known to be one of the smartest game fish.

The life cycle of the bass starts in the spring. The spawning male bass heads for shallow water, and there he clears an area for a nest. He uses his tail to fan the lake bed and remove all loose sand and particles until the grass roots in the lake bottom appear.

A female bass joins him. She is usually much larger than the male. When the clearing is finished, the female lays her eggs and the male fertilizes them.

Then the male takes over protecting the eggs. He even chases the female away from the nest, for females often eat their own eggs. When his nest is threatened, he will attack an enemy many times his size. Sunfish and other fish can "smell" the eggs and rush in to eat them. Often, while the bass is busy chasing one sunfish away, another sunfish rushes in and helps itself to the eggs.

1. This selection mostly talks about
   □ a. different kinds of fresh water fish.
   □ b. bass fishing.
   □ c. the life cycle of the bass.
   □ d. stocking fresh water lakes.

2. For most animals living is
   □ a. mostly play with a little work.
   □ b. an easy chore.
   □ c. boring and uninteresting.
   □ d. a constant life and death struggle.

3. Female bass
   □ a. often eat their own eggs.
   □ b. feed on sunfish.
   □ c. fertilize the eggs.
   □ d. are smaller than the male.

4. Many animals never die of old age because
   □ a. animals never age.
   □ b. most of the time they die of disease.
   □ c. they are usually killed by another animal.
   □ d. animals have strong hearts.

5. A "weedy" swamp is filled with many
   □ a. insects.
   □ b. animals.
   □ c. plants.
   □ d. rocks.

6. When a nest is <u>threatened</u> it is
   □ a. not well built.
   □ b. untidy.
   □ c. well made.
   □ d. in danger.

CATEGORIES OF COMPREHENSION QUESTIONS

No. 1: Subject Matter	No. 3: Supporting Details	No. 5: Clarifying Devices
No. 2: Main Idea	No. 4: Conclusion	No. 6: Vocabulary in Context

5. THE HUNTER AND THE HUNTED

If the male bass has succeeded in protecting the eggs, they will hatch three or four days after being laid. Then the tiny bass will head for the brownish-green grass where there is more protection. Each will be about a quarter of an inch long and will swarm around their father like bees.

In two or three weeks, the little fry will grow into 2-inch *fingerlings*. But out of hundreds hatched, only a few dozen are left. The rest have been eaten by other larger fish.

When the young bass are about three weeks old, the father will leave them, and the fingerlings scatter to find food. Completely on their own, they must learn to watch out for sunfish, pickerel, carp and other bass, including their own parents.

The fingerlings will start eating by nibbling at insect larvae. As they grow, they will become meat-eating hunters in their own right. Their already wide mouths will grow wider. They will terrorize the smaller fish around them. As hunters, they may eat crayfish, snakes, sunfish, bluefish, other smaller bass and even ducklings and baby muskrats!

A full-grown bass may weigh 10 to 15 pounds, but a few will grow to 25 pounds and measure 3 feet in length. The smartest and strongest among them will go on growing and hunting until they are twenty years old. Some scientists believe they would go on living for many more years except that the killer is killed, either by disease or a smarter, faster enemy from another environment. From above the water an air-breathing mammal, such as the otter, may enter the watery world at any time and take the bass for food.

So the hunter becomes the prey, but the life cycle of the bass again repeats itself in the little fry he has left behind.

1. This article is about
   ☐ a. bass.
   ☐ b. pickerel.
   ☐ c. carp.
   ☐ d. sunfish.

2. The writer's main idea is that
   ☐ a. fresh water fish are tasty.
   ☐ b. fish live a long time.
   ☐ c. small fish live in the grass for protection.
   ☐ d. the life cycle repeats itself.

3. Fingerlings feed on
   ☐ a. fish eggs.
   ☐ b. insect larvae.
   ☐ c. grassy plants.
   ☐ d. algae.

4. When a fish first hatches, it is called a
   ☐ a. pup.
   ☐ b. fry.
   ☐ c. fingerling.
   ☐ d. yearling.

5. A "full-grown" bass is
   ☐ a. an egg.
   ☐ b. a baby.
   ☐ c. an adult.
   ☐ d. a young female.

6. A terrorized fish is
   ☐ a. angry.
   ☐ b. frightened.
   ☐ c. quarrelsome.
   ☐ d. shy.

CATEGORIES OF COMPREHENSION QUESTIONS

| No. 1: Subject Matter | No. 3: Supporting Details | No. 5: Clarifying Devices |
| No. 2: Main Idea | No. 4· Conclusion | No. 6: Vocabulary in Context |

6. THE HOLDER OF SOIL AND WATER

Before man plowed the land, grass mixed with other plants covered much of the earth. Dead plants built up a fertile layer of soil called *humus*. A network of roots grew down into the soil. Each one made a tiny channel through which rain ran into the earth. Spongy layers of stems, leaves and roots soaked up falling rain so that it could not wash the soil away.

Then man discovered that he could plant seeds and grow crops. He began to plow the earth and remove the natural cover. The unprotected soil that had been beneath this cover blew and washed away.

Soil became damaged or *eroded* so badly that some ancient civilizations disappeared. For instance, northern Mongolia was once a rich land. But it was overgrazed by too many sheep and became a wasteland. The history of man is full of such examples of bad land use.

In the United States, millions of acres of land were plowed to make farms. The land was also overgrazed by too many cattle. Some of the land eroded so badly that it became useless. Water dug gulleys into the soil, and wind blew soil away. During the 1920s and early 1930s, soil blew away in great clouds, wiping out whole farms and burying the buildings.

After the dry years in the United States from 1925 to 1932, the whole nation became alarmed about soil erosion. So Congress set up the United States Soil Conservation Service as part of the Department of Agriculture. Scientists in this department worked with farmers and ranchers to restore the soil. They planted drainage channels with covers of living grass. They limited the number of animals that could graze on natural rangelands so the grass could grow again and many farmers began to grow a new cover of soil-holding grass.

1. This passage is about
   ☐ a. fertilization.
   ☐ b. crop rotation.
   ☐ c. soil erosion.
   ☐ d. irrigation.

2. The best soil-holder is
   ☐ a. grass.
   ☐ b. shrubbery.
   ☐ c. cultivated crops.
   ☐ d. the small rodent family.

3. The dry years in the United States came
   ☐ a. between 1800 and 1860.
   ☐ b. between 1920 and 1930.
   ☐ c. between 1940 and 1950.
   ☐ d. between 1955 and 1960.

4. According to this article, soil becomes damaged by all of the following except
   ☐ a. wind.   ☐ c. water.
   ☐ b. overgrazing.   ☐ d. fertilizer.

5. Spongy plants
   ☐ a. soak up water.
   ☐ b. are tough.
   ☐ c. can be troublesome.
   ☐ d. bend easily.

6. As used in this article, <u>alarmed</u> means
   ☐ a. bored.
   ☐ b. sarcastic.
   ☐ c. concerned.
   ☐ d. useless.

CATEGORIES OF COMPREHENSION QUESTIONS

No. 1: Subject Matter   No. 3: Supporting Details   No. 5: Clarifying Devices
No. 2: Main Idea   No. 4: Conclusion   No. 6: Vocabulary in Context

7. THE GRAY BIRCH – I

The little seed from the gray birch was only about the size of the o's on this page. It had come loose, with many others like it, from the old tree which grew at the edge of the forest next to an abandoned cornfield. A sudden wind had bent and shaken the tall white trunk of the birch. Now the seed was sailing far out over the field, carried along by two little wings.

Other kinds of seeds had been blown from their parent trees by the same wind. But the seeds of the oak, beech and hickory trees were heavy nuts and didn't have wings to carry them into the field. They had fallen to the forest floor a few feet from their parent trees.

The gust of wind carrying the little birch seed began losing strength. Suddenly the seed was falling! Below it the cornfield was a jungle of grasses and other plants that had begun to grow soon after the farmer had moved.

The tiny seed fell under a blackberry bush, where it was quiet and shadowy. A few days later a light snowfall covered the gray birch seed. All winter it lay quietly under the snow.

The early spring sun coming through the blackberry stems cast long shadows on the melting snow. It took several days of warm weather to start the little seed growing. It sent tiny white roots into the dark soil where there should have been water and minerals. But there was little mineral nourishment in the soil of the old field. Most of it had been used up by the corn which had grown there for many years. Other kinds of tree seedlings would have died in such poor soil, but not the gray birch!

Within a few months the seed had become a young tree. The farmer probably wouldn't have thought of it as a tree because its trunk was just about the thickness of a pencil lead, and it had only eight leaves. These green leaves were making food for the tree whenever the sun shone. They made the food out of carbon dioxide from the air and water brought up by the roots. This is called photosynthesis (fo to SIN thuh sis).

Time passed, and on its first birthday the little tree was already pushing its way up through the prickly stems of the blackberry bush. On its third birthday the gray birch was taller than the bush!

Every birthday that followed found the gray birch taller. By its tenth birthday its trunk was about as thick as the handle of a baseball bat. The bark changed to a grayish-white with V-shaped marks.

1. Select the best title.
 □ a. Birth of a Tree
 □ b. How to Tell a Tree's Age
 □ c. Bears and Birch Trees
 □ d. Poems about Trees

2. Birch trees
 □ a. have a difficult time growing in wet soil.
 □ b. grow from very small seeds that sprout in the spring.
 □ c. become heavy with nuts.
 □ d. seem to grow best in salt marshes.

3. The food making process of green-leafed plants is called
 □ a. photographic.
 □ b. photoelectric.
 □ c. phototropic.
 □ d. photosynthesis.

4. It seems that birch trees
 □ a. do not need soil that is rich in minerals.
 □ b. are easily killed by too much snow.
 □ c. do not lose their leaves in winter.
 □ d. have exploding seeds.

5. A "jungle of grasses" means the grass is
 □ a. a tropical kind.
 □ b. useful.
 □ c. very thick.
 □ d. well watered.

6. As used in this passage, nourishment is
 □ a. wind.
 □ b. carbon dioxide.
 □ c. food.
 □ d. sunlight.

CATEGORIES OF COMPREHENSION QUESTIONS

No. 1: Subject Matter   No. 3: Supporting Details   No. 5: Clarifying Devices
No. 2: Main Idea   No. 4: Conclusion   No. 6: Vocabulary in Context

8. THE GRAY BIRCH — II

Each spring shiny green leaves shaped like triangles popped out from buds on the twigs. In a summer wind, they fluttered and danced on long stems. When autumn came, the leaves turned a deep golden color. The birch's leaves which fell each autumn, together with the leaves of the other plants growing around it, slowly built up a thin layer of rich soil.

One fall day, when the birch was about twelve years old (that's almost middle age for a gray birch), a squirrel buried an acorn in the ground under the tree. The squirrel intended to come back for the acorn but forgot it.

After a time the acorn began to grow. It used minerals from the layer of rich soil that the birch and the other plants had laid down on top of the once bare soil. The leaves of the birch shaded the oak seedling from the hot sun.

The oak's growing close by didn't bother the birch for many years. But one spring, after the birch had flowered and opened its leaves, it had trouble getting enough sunlight to make its food. The oak had grown so tall that now its leaves kept the sun from reaching the birch.

The next winter was a very hard one for all the birches. Heavy wet snow and thick coats of ice made them bend way over until their top branches almost touched the ground. When it was younger, the gray birch would have sprung back up again when the snow and ice melted, but not this time! Somewhere in its thick trunk something had snapped. That spring the birch could straighten up only slightly.

Later, insects were able to enter the weakened old tree. Inside the trunk, they and their offspring ate away at the birch. It was also weakened by the woodpeckers that came to dig out the insects. They picked with their sharp bills and made a loud clatter.

The tiny seedlike spores of a fungus were carried to the tree by the wind. They entered the trunk through openings made by the insects and sent out long thin threads into the wood. The fungus used the wood for food, too.

That winter a big storm toppled the gray birch to the ground. Snow covered it and rain fell upon it. Now other kinds of insects and fungi lived in the wood and used it for food. What was left gradually became part of the soil. Overhead the oak would continue to grow for many more years, thanks to the birch.

1. This story tells about
   ☐ a. gray birch seedlings.
   ☐ b. the roots and bark of a gray birch.
   ☐ c. the death of a gray birch.
   ☐ d. how gray birches get food.

2. The gray birch's problems started with
   ☐ a. wood-eating insects.
   ☐ b. lack of water.
   ☐ c. a fungus that attacked its bark.
   ☐ d. the growth of a small oak.

3. Each autumn the leaves of the birch became
   ☐ a. a deep gold.
   ☐ b. green.
   ☐ c. a brilliant red.
   ☐ d. orange.

4. Rotting leaves
   ☐ a. can kill oak seedlings.
   ☐ b. poison the soil.
   ☐ c. add iron to the soil.
   ☐ d. make the soil rich.

5. The woodpeckers that came to the birch were
   ☐ a. quiet.
   ☐ b. playful.
   ☐ c. noisy.
   ☐ d. bashful.

6. A seedling is a
   ☐ a. bush.
   ☐ b. tree's trunk.
   ☐ c. fungus.
   ☐ d. young tree.

CATEGORIES OF COMPREHENSION QUESTIONS

No. 1: Subject Matter   No. 3: Supporting Details   No. 5: Clarifying Devices
No. 2: Main Idea   No. 4: Conclusion   No. 6: Vocabulary in Context

---

9. THE HOT-COLD DESERT

The desert! Who would want to go to the desert — that hot, barren, sandy wasteland? That's the way many people describe the desert. But we shall see that the desert is one of the most interesting habitats on this entire planet. Once you discover its <u>endless</u> beauty and peace, you will want to return again and again.

Deserts are very hot because the air is so dry and clear that the sun's light comes through more strongly. In summer the sun beats down furiously. This turns the land into a radiator, which, like the radiator in your house, heats the air which touches it. One July day in Death Valley, the desert temperature went up to 134° F. The land itself might be as hot as 180° F. At that temperature you'd better not touch it!

But take a sweater with you when you visit the desert! Heat escapes very quickly through the moisture-free air. Soon after sunset the air cools and you will feel chilly.

Have you wondered why pictures of Arabs show them wearing many clothes during the hot desert day? Lightweight, light-colored garments insulate their bodies against heat during the day and from the cold at night.

When winter comes, many deserts are delightful places to live. Palm Springs, California, and Tucson, Arizona, are favorite winter vacation areas in the United States. Some northern or "cold" deserts, such as those in Utah and Wyoming, have plenty of cold winter weather with some snow and ice.

The desert, then, is not always hot, but it is usually dry because it gets so little rain or snow. When you are in the southern Arizona desert and you wash your hands, they almost become dry before you can reach for your towel. Sometimes when it rains only lightly, you can see the rain falling, but it disappears before it reaches the ground. The raindrops evaporate as they fall.

1. This article is mostly about desert
   □ a. plants.
   □ b. animals.
   □ c. people.
   □ d. temperatures.

2. The desert is one of the most
   □ a. colorful habitats in the world.
   □ b. unattractive land forms on earth.
   □ c. interesting places on this planet.
   □ d. common wastelands on earth.

3. The desert nights are
   □ a. windy.
   □ b. cool.
   □ c. hot.
   □ d. long.

4. This article hints that all deserts are
   □ a. hot.
   □ b. dry.
   □ c. sandy.
   □ d. wastelands.

5. In the first paragraph the writer is trying to explain how most people
   □ a. live on the desert.
   □ b. enjoy the desert.
   □ c. travel on the desert.
   □ d. describe the desert.

6. Endless beauty
   □ a. lasts forever.
   □ b. is seasonal.
   □ c. changes rapidly.
   □ d. is man-made.

CATEGORIES OF COMPREHENSION QUESTIONS

No. 1: Subject Matter   No. 3: Supporting Details   No. 5: Clarifying Devices
No. 2: Main Idea   No. 4: Conclusion   No. 6: Vocabulary in Context

---

10. ARE ALL DESERTS SANDY?

Scientists decided long ago that areas with generally high temperatures and an average rainfall amounting to less than 10 inches a year are deserts. In some years, if you lived in the Nevada desert, you might collect only 3 or 4 inches of rain per year, whereas other deserts might have 12 or 13.

When a heavy rain does come to the desert, the dry soil cannot soak up the water fast enough. Unable to soak into the ground, the pouring rain flows toward dry stream beds called *arroyos*. These quickly become raging rivers. Since most deserts are in low areas covering hundreds of square miles, water flows toward them rather than toward the sea. This creates temporary lakes. Occasionally large lakes are formed such as the Great Salt Lake in Utah.

As the water evaporates, large mineral deposits are left. Death Valley developed huge stores of borax this way. The salt flats of Utah are rich in common salt and in potash, which is mined for fertilizer.

How will your body feel if you spend some time in the desert? In summer you will feel hot from midmorning to sunset. If heat bothers you, stay in the shade of your car, tent or even under a picnic table. You will perspire several quarts of water as your body cools itself, but the air is so dry that you will not feel sweaty. Whether you feel thirsty or not, *drink something every hour*. Otherwise, dehydration sickness (loss of water) will spoil your fun for awhile. Illness can also result when perspiring removes your body's salt. It's a good idea to salt your food well or take salt <u>tablets</u>.

Would a desert be complete without plenty of sand? Some deserts, such as the Sahara and Arabian, have mile upon mile of sand dunes. In our own American deserts, however, you will need to look hard for the sandy deserts like those you see on television. Most of the loose sand was blown or washed away long ago. The pebbles and stones left behind form an odd "pavement."

1. Choose the best title.
   - ☐ a. Animals of the Desert
   - ☐ b. Water and the Desert
   - ☐ c. Plants and Desert Life
   - ☐ d. Nomads of the Sahara

2. According to this passage, a desert has
   - ☐ a. high temperatures and little rain.
   - ☐ b. many different kinds of plants and animals.
   - ☐ c. many aluminum deposits.
   - ☐ d. a mixture of nomadic people.

3. Dehydration sickness results from
   - ☐ a. eating spoiled food.
   - ☐ b. wearing too many warm clothes.
   - ☐ c. drinking too much water.
   - ☐ d. a great loss of body water.

4. We can guess that not all deserts
   - ☐ a. have plants.
   - ☐ b. are dry.
   - ☐ c. are sandy.
   - ☐ d. are rich in minerals.

5. A "raging river" looks very
   - ☐ a. clever.
   - ☐ b. angry.
   - ☐ c. bashful.
   - ☐ d. friendly.

6. As used in this selection, a salt tablet is
   - ☐ a. a wall panel.
   - ☐ b. a game.
   - ☐ c. writing paper.
   - ☐ d. a flat disk.

CATEGORIES OF COMPREHENSION QUESTIONS

No. 1: Subject Matter	No. 3: Supporting Details	No. 5: Clarifying Devices
No. 2: Main Idea	No. 4: Conclusion	No. 6: Vocabulary in Context

11. MIGHTY MOOSE

In order to feed its enormous body, the moose eats 35 pounds of food a day. It strips the leaves and twigs from many kinds of trees. It eats bark and lichens. Going into the water, it clips off floating water lilies and duckweed. It scoops up underwater bur reed and duck potato. Small wonder that the Algonquin Indians named this great American elk "musee" or "twig-eater." Twig-eating is called "browsing."

Browsing keeps the huge mammal on the go. This workout is a must, for a moose's digestion is easily upset. Moose kept in zoos get sick because they cannot exercise. Without proper diet and activity they cannot survive. Moose feed mornings and evenings, so these are good times to watch them if you can. In spite of its size, a moose can move through the forest in almost complete silence when it wants to. At other times, it crashes through like a bulldozer.

It's hard to mistake the huge, sway-backed moose for any other animal. It has a droopy, oversized <u>muzzle</u> and long, floppy ears. A hairy strip of skin dangles from its throat. This 4- to 10-inch strip is called a "bell" or "dewlap."

When autumn brings snow to the mountains and lakes freeze over, moose seek food in lower country. Moose are not very sociable. However, in winter several animals band together or "yard up." Moose are active even in the most severe weather. Their long legs and spreading hooves help them get through the snow.

Hungry wolves stalk and kill the young and the sick moose. A healthy moose does not panic at the sight of its natural enemy. If attacked, it can fight off a pack of wolves with its powerful forefeet. If forced into flight, it can outrun wolves through soft, deep snow. But if the snow is crusted over, the wolves have the advantage of being able to run on top while the moose breaks through and flounders.

The mighty moose leave their yards in the spring. Bulls move on to higher country while cows go their separate ways to find calving places where their young will be born. A calf's bay-colored, unspotted coat is much lighter than that of its mother. It does not yet have a shoulder hump or drooping upper lip, but it does have its parents' sharp sense of smell and hearing.

The long-legged calf soon stands up and follows its mother. She teaches it swimming, browsing and self-defense. Sometimes a calf stays with its mother until she has another calf the following spring.

Our mighty moose live in wilderness areas from Maine to Alaska and south through the Rocky Mountains to Wyoming.

1. Another title for this selection would be
   □ a. Defenses of the Moose.
   □ b. "Musee" the Great American Elk.
   □ c. Moose and Reindeer.
   □ d. Moose Fossils for Sale.

2. The writer's main point is
   □ a. to explain the reasons for hunting moose.
   □ b. to show how the moose uses its sense of smell.
   □ c. to describe how animal fossils form.
   □ d. to discuss many facts about the moose.

3. Each day, an adult moose will eat
   □ a. 5 pounds of food.
   □ b. 15 pounds of food.
   □ c. 20 pounds of food.
   □ d. 35 pounds of food.

4. We can see that the moose usually
   □ a. does well in captivity.
   □ b. has an unfriendly nature.
   □ c. is found in herds.
   □ d. makes a good work animal.

5. A calf has a bay-colored coat. This means its coat is
   □ a. black.
   □ b. pure white.
   □ c. reddish brown.
   □ d. brown and white.

6. A moose's muzzle is its
   □ a. tongue.
   □ b. lip.
   □ c. chin.
   □ d. nose.

CATEGORIES OF COMPREHENSION QUESTIONS

No. 1: Subject Matter   No. 3: Supporting Details   No. 5: Clarifying Devices
No. 2: Main Idea   No. 4: Conclusion   No. 6: Vocabulary in Context

---

12. SNAILS

What animal walks on one foot, has a mouth like a file, a body twisted like a screw and though it never makes a sound, always leaves a trail? A snail!

There are both land and water snails. Land snails have lungs and breathe air. Most water snails have gills, somewhat like those of a fish, which get oxygen from the water. Some water snails have lungs and must come to the surface to breathe air through a tube that serves as a built-in snorkel. Many can even leave the water and move about on land.

Land snails are common in the woods. However, you won't find them in evergreen forests because the soil is too acidy. Most stay hidden in the soil or under fallen trees or decaying leaves. They are often the same color as the soil or leaves.

Because their bodies must be kept moist, snails usually stay in the shade, but on cloudy, damp days, you may find one searching for food in the open.

Water snails can be found clinging to plants and rocks in almost any body of water. Since the water prevents them from drying out, they can be found moving about all through the day.

Don't be afraid to pick up a snail — it can't bite. While you're holding the snail, look at its shell. The snail carries its home around on its back and can pull back into its shell for protection against many enemies. Also, when its surroundings get cold or dry, it can pull inside and sleep.

Its shell always grows in a spiral. It grows around and around, getting bigger as it turns. As the animal grows, it makes a larger shell.

When the snail pokes out of its shell, look at it. It won't be afraid of you, because it doesn't really "see" as you do. Most snails can see only if there is a change in the light.

On the bottom of the snail's body is its mouth. It has a file-like tongue called a *radula* (RAJ oo luh) which is covered with many tiny teeth. It uses this radula to scrape small bits of food into its mouth.

Another part on the bottom of its body is its traveling pad, called its "foot." Set the snail down on something and it seems to just flow along like a snake. It doesn't have any legs and doesn't need any. Put it on a pane of glass and watch it from the other side. You will soon see muscular waves pass down its foot, carrying the snail forward. It helps itself by secreting slime which makes it easier to slide along.

1. Choose the best title.
   - ☐ a. Facts about Snails
   - ☐ b. Snails and Shellfish
   - ☐ c. The Damaging Snail
   - ☐ d. The Snail — A Special Treat

2. The writer tells us there are
   - ☐ a. no snails in North America.
   - ☐ b. some very dangerous snails.
   - ☐ c. snails that make good pets.
   - ☐ d. both land and water snails.

3. Snails must keep their bodies
   - ☐ a. clean.
   - ☐ b. dry.
   - ☐ c. moist.
   - ☐ d. oiled.

4. Snails are
   - ☐ a. harmless.
   - ☐ d. curious.
   - ☐ c. tricky.
   - ☐ d. noisy.

5. A "spiral shell" is shaped like
   - ☐ a. a saw.
   - ☐ b. a wrench.
   - ☐ c. a screw.
   - ☐ d. a hammer.

6. Decaying leaves are
   - ☐ a. interesting leaves.
   - ☐ b. moving leaves.
   - ☐ c. budding leaves.
   - ☐ d. rotting leaves.

CATEGORIES OF COMPREHENSION QUESTIONS

No. 1: Subject Matter	No. 3: Supporting Details	No. 5: Clarifying Devices
No. 2: Main Idea	No. 4: Conclusion	No. 6: Vocabulary in Context

13. ON THE TRAIL OF THE SNAIL

Snails are great animals to watch. Most are small, so they don't need a big cage. They're slow, so they can't get away quickly. They can't bite and they don't have a bad odor.

The snail won't be frightened if you talk — it can't hear. What disturbs it is to be touched.

You can keep a land snail in a jar with one or two holes in the lid. It has to have air, but be sure the holes aren't so big that it can get out — it can climb right up the straight sides of a jar.

Put some soil from the place where you found the snail into the jar. About an inch is enough. A piece of bark or some wet dead leaves can go over the soil. Add a stick for your snail to climb on. You can even grow a little plant or two in the jar if there is room. Keep the soil damp, but be careful — too much water can drown a land snail.

A water snail can be kept in a jar nearly filled with water taken from the same place where you found the snail. Some get their oxygen from air; others get it from the water.

Punch holes in the jar above the water level so air can get to the water. Place a few water plants and algae-covered rocks in the jar. These will give off oxygen and provide food for your snail. If you have an aquarium, you probably have some pond snails in it. They help clean the aquarium.

Most land snails eat live or dead plants. To find out what kind of food your snail likes, first offer it tiny bits of different foods. Some snails like leafy food, such as lettuce. Others like fruit, such as apples. A few kinds even like a bit of raw hamburger. Offer a flake of raw oatmeal or wheat cereal, even a cracker crumb. If it doesn't eat the food after a few hours, be sure to take it away before it spoils.

Don't be surprised if your snail "glues" itself to the side of the jar or under the lid. Most land and fresh-water snails hibernate part of the year, so just let yours sleep.

You can always safely turn your pet loose where you found it, so long as the weather is not too cold. It will go about its business just as it did before you picked it up.

1. Another good title would be
   □ a. What about a Pet Snail?
   □ b. Snails of the Tropics.
   □ c. Snails Are Good for Your Garden.
   □ d. Ever Eat Snails?

2. Snails are
   □ a. hard to find.
   □ b. disturbed by noise.
   □ c. great fun to watch.
   □ d. fairly large animals.

3. Pond snails are good for your aquarium because they
   □ a. are food for the other fish.
   □ b. help keep it clean.
   □ c. add oxygen to the water.
   □ d. take up very little room.

4. The oxygen in water probably comes from
   □ a. sunlight.
   □ b. rocks.
   □ c. fish.
   □ d. water plants.

5. The seventh paragraph talks about
   □ a. the snail's shell.
   □ b. mating habits of the snail.
   □ c. water snails.
   □ d. the snail's diet.

6. Raw oatmeal has not been
   □ a. packaged.
   □ b. cooked.
   □ c. refrigerated.
   □ d. salted.

CATEGORIES OF COMPREHENSION QUESTIONS

No. 1: Subject Matter   No. 3: Supporting Details   No. 5: Clarifying Devices
No. 2: Main Idea   No. 4: Conclusion   No. 6: Vocabulary in Context

14. PEANUTS ANYONE?

Who likes peanuts more than elephants do? People do! We eat them in many forms. We cook with peanut oil. We make a number of things with peanuts from plastics to cattle food to candy.

You may think that you already know a lot about the peanut, but our nutty friend is full of surprises. To begin with, it tastes like a nut and is used like a nut, but it is not a nut at all! It is the seed of a plant belonging to the *pea* family. The clue is in its name: PEA-nut.

All plants have *some* way of making sure their seeds find places to grow. Usually they depend on outside help, such as the wind or rain. Not the peanut — it plants its own seeds!

A raw peanut sprouts and sends up leaves and stems. Soon it becomes a plant about a foot or more in height. Before long this busy plant is covered with bright yellow blossoms.

After fertilizing themselves, the flowers wither and fall off. The stems where the flowers were attached, which are called *pegs*, begin to grow longer and longer. The pegs curve downward as they grow, pushing their tips a few inches into the ground. The tiny seeds inside the tips slowly grow and begin forming peanuts. The tips of the stems become the peanut shells or pods. Not only are the plant's seeds well protected, but they are ready to sprout into new little peanut plants the following spring.

When the old plants die in the fall, harvesters dig them up along with the seeds. Then either the pods are stripped off and sent to market or they are opened and the seeds are removed. The empty pods are ground up and used as a soil conditioner.

Although peanuts have been widely known as food for hundreds of years, one man is responsible for discovering that the peanut had many other uses. His name was George Washington Carver. As a boy, he was poor, but he worked his way through school and finally college. Eventually he became one of the world's most famous botanists and agricultural chemists.

Mr. Carver was able to show people how to make over 300 different products from peanuts and peanut hulls. These range from ink to "instant coffee" to soap.

Peanuts contain many vitamins and minerals as well as protein. So, the peanut which is so useful and so tasty, especially as peanut butter, is also good for you.

1. This article tells us
   ☐ a. many facts about the peanut.
   ☐ b. how peanuts are roasted.
   ☐ c. the history of the peanut.
   ☐ d. why people dislike peanuts.

2. The peanut is
   ☐ a. a kind of nut.
   ☐ b. related to squash.
   ☐ c. surprisingly useful.
   ☐ d. often killed by frost.

3. The man that discovered much about the peanut was
   ☐ a. Alexander Graham Bell.
   ☐ b. Louis Pasteur.
   ☐ c. Thomas Edison.
   ☐ d. George Washington Carver.

4. The peanut shells are
   ☐ a. moist and often swollen.
   ☐ b. used to protect the seed.
   ☐ c. soft and wet.
   ☐ d. easily damaged.

5. Empty pods are "ground up." This means they have been
   ☐ a. dried and are being stored.
   ☐ b. buried.
   ☐ c. mixed with soil.
   ☐ d. broken into very small pieces.

6. A clue is a
   ☐ a. fact.
   ☐ b. number.
   ☐ c. hint.
   ☐ d. seed.

CATEGORIES OF COMPREHENSION QUESTIONS		
No. 1: Subject Matter	No. 3: Supporting Details	No. 5: Clarifying Devices
No. 2: Main Idea	No. 4: Conclusion	No. 6: Vocabulary in Context

15. JET-PROPELLED SCALLOPS

Do you know that some mollusks used jet propulsion millions of years before planes zoomed through the sky? They still are doing it.

If, on a summer's night, you stand on a rocky sea shore, you might hear a soft clickety-clack sound. You might worry about what it is, but don't.

The clickety-clack is probably being made by *Pecten irradians* jetting along the surface of the ocean water. The name sounds as if it belongs to some sort of sea monster, but it is just a small, harmless creature known as a bay or common scallop.

The scallop shell is truly "scalloped." About nineteen ridges fan out from a flat hinge at the back of the shell.

When first taken from the sea, a scallop shell is dull blackish-brown on the outside and milky-white inside. When it dries, beautiful soft shades of yellow, orange, red or sometimes purple may appear inside.

The female bay scallop lays about two million eggs that quickly hatch. The young scallops, called "spats," attach themselves to blades of eel grass, submerged plant life or sunken objects. The ever-changing tides bring a great deal of microscopic life to feed the spats.

When the spat reaches about 1-1/2 inches in size, it detaches itself. It can now swim by jet propulsion. It has a big muscle at the hinge where its two shells are joined. It can open the shells to take in water. By squeezing the shells together, it can force the water out two small openings near the hinge. This shoots the creature through the water in any direction at a good speed. As the scallop does this, the edges of its shell vibrate, making a clickety-clack like the sound of a small engine. The hinge muscle is about an inch thick. It varies in size from that of a penny to that of a nickel. The muscle is considered very good to eat.

1. This passage is mainly about how scallops
   - ☐ a. move.
   - ☐ b. mate.
   - ☐ c. grow.
   - ☐ d. raise their young.

2. The main thought of this selection is
   - ☐ a. mollusks have soft bodies.
   - ☐ b. scallops have used jet propulsion for millions of years.
   - ☐ c. jet propulsion is harmful.
   - ☐ d. scallops are colorful but dangerous to touch.

3. Young scallops are called
   - ☐ a. gems.
   - ☐ b. larvae.
   - ☐ c. nymphs.
   - ☐ d. spats.

4. The writer suggests that in order to use jet propulsion the scallop must have a strong
   - ☐ a. muscle.
   - ☐ b. shell.
   - ☐ c. foot.
   - ☐ d. mouth.

5. Ever-changing tides are
   - ☐ a. very weak.
   - ☐ b. never still.
   - ☐ c. not too large.
   - ☐ d. quiet and calm.

6. Submerged plant life is found
   - ☐ a. on rocks.
   - ☐ b. underwater.
   - ☐ c. in caves.
   - ☐ d. in deserts.

CATEGORIES OF COMPREHENSION QUESTIONS

No. 1: Subject Matter   No. 3: Supporting Details   No. 5: Clarifying Devices
No. 2: Main Idea   No. 4: Conclusion   No. 6: Vocabulary in Context

16. HARVESTING THE SCALLOP

Inside the shell the soft body of the scallop has a fleshy covering called the mantle. This provides thin layers of shell material as the scallop grows. On the edge of the mantle is a row of beautiful iridescent dots, bright blue in color. These are called its "eyes." They do seem to be sensitive to light, but it is believed that the scallop is not able to see through them.

When the scallop passes the immature stage, it is ready to settle down on the ocean floor. It can be found in thick strands of eel grass or other marine growth. It "walks" on the bottom by pushing itself along with a sort of muscular foot that sticks out from between its shells.

Bay scallops are gathered by fishermen using dredge nets. These nets look something like a large purse with the top open. They are dragged along the ocean floor by boats. A lone fisherman will usually use only one dredge, but some boats can drag up to six if there is extra help aboard.

Every so often the dredge is hauled aboard the boat and the contents dumped on the deck. The scallops are picked out and put in bags. Most of the rest of the haul is put back into the sea. Starfish and whelks that are caught are destroyed because they eat the scallops.

Finally, the scallops are brought to shore and opened to get at the edible muscle. The rest of the scallops' "innards" are thrown into the water where the ever-hungry gulls gobble them down. The shells are ground or broken up for use in making roads.

The scallop's shell design has been popular for many centuries. If you look around, you are sure to see it as part of a decoration somewhere. One large oil company uses it as its symbol.

I hope someday you may enjoy a delicious meal of fresh bay scallops. When you do, remember: You are eating part of one of the world's oldest jets!

1. The scallop is a
   - ☐ a. goldfish.
   - ☐ b. shellfish.
   - ☐ c. starfish.
   - ☐ d. sunfish.

2. Bay scallops are gathered by using
   - ☐ a. fish hooks.
   - ☐ b. sea worms.
   - ☐ c. lobster pots.
   - ☐ d. dredge nets.

3. The scallop walks by using its
   - ☐ a. muscular foot.
   - ☐ b. shell.
   - ☐ c. eyes.
   - ☐ d. mantle.

4. A natural enemy of the scallop is the
   - ☐ a. starfish.
   - ☐ b. sand shark.
   - ☐ c. octopus.
   - ☐ d. moray eel.

5. A "fleshy covering" would feel
   - ☐ a. soft.
   - ☐ b. cold.
   - ☐ c. bumpy.
   - ☐ d. brittle.

6. An immature scallop is a
   - ☐ a. well-hidden scallop.
   - ☐ b. tough scallop.
   - ☐ c. young scallop.
   - ☐ d. weak scallop.

CATEGORIES OF COMPREHENSION QUESTIONS

| No. 1: Subject Matter | No. 3: Supporting Details | No. 5: Clarifying Devices |
| No. 2: Main Idea | No. 4: Conclusion | No. 6: Vocabulary in Context |

17. STARS OF THE SEA

Starfish are animals, but they don't *look* very animal-like. Starfish eat shellfish such as clams, mussels, oysters and scallops.

When a starfish finds a shellfish, it drapes itself over its victim. The starfish holds on tightly with its "tube feet" and pulls the two shells apart. The starfish isn't very strong, but it can keep up a steady pull for a long, long time. Sooner or later, the shellfish must relax the muscle holding the shells together, and so let them open.

The mouth of the starfish is located in the center of the underside where the arms join. The starfish pushes its own stomach out through its mouth and into the shellfish! Digestion takes place completely outside the starfish's body. The digested food is taken into the stomach. Then the stomach is pulled back inside the starfish.

Man likes to eat shellfish, too. Fishermen gather shellfish to sell in the markets. So the starfish competes with the fishermen. Actually, starfish cost the shellfishing industry many thousands of dollars every year, perhaps even millions!

The fishermen work hard to catch and remove all the starfish that get into their favorite shellfishing beds and the "underwater farms" where they raise clams and oysters. They used to haul the starfish into their boats, chop them in two with axes or knives and throw the pieces overboard. They thought this would get rid of the starfish. What they didn't know was that *each piece* of the cut-up starfish, if it's big enough, will grow into a whole new animal! When the fishermen cut up 100 starfish and threw the halves overboard, they actually made 200 new starfish! Today they keep the starfish in their boats and throw them ashore where they quickly dry out and die.

The starfish is not really a "fish." Its close relatives are sea urchins, basket stars, brittle stars, sea cucumbers and sea lilies. They have all lived successfully on the earth for many billions of years. They live in both shallow water and at the bottom of the ocean, some at a depth of 27,000 feet. With their ability to survive, starfish will probably go on their merry way for many centuries to come.

1. Starfish are
   □ a. reptiles.
   □ b. fish.
   □ c. animals.
   □ d. mammals.

2. Starfish eat
   □ a. other starfish.
   □ b. plankton.
   □ c. small fish.
   □ d. shellfish.

3. Starfish have been found at depths of
   □ a. 27,000 feet.
   □ b. 50,000 feet.
   □ c. 75,000 feet.
   □ d. 97,000 feet.

4. We can see that starfish cannot live
   □ a. in thick areas of seaweed.
   □ b. out of water.
   □ c. in shallow water.
   □ d. underwater.

5. Fishermen find starfish
   □ a. a problem.
   □ b. good eating.
   □ c. a big help to the fishing industry.
   □ d. enjoyable creatures.

6. As used in this article, <u>relax</u> means to
   □ a. hold tight.
   □ b. eat.
   □ c. swim.
   □ d. loosen.

CATEGORIES OF COMPREHENSION QUESTIONS

No. 1: Subject Matter	No. 3: Supporting Details	No. 5: Clarifying Devices
No. 2: Main Idea	No. 4: Conclusion	No. 6: Vocabulary in Context

18. TRAVELING SEEDS

Most traveling seeds go by air. When you blow off a dandelion's fluffy white head, you are doing just what the wind does — spreading its seeds. Dandelion and milkweed seeds are attached to silky parachutes that help carry them through the air. Cottonwood seeds are covered with fine hairs that help them fly through the air.

Maple, elm and many pine seeds are like little helicopters. They have wings that whirl in the wind, carrying them far from the parent trees.

There are seeds so small and light that they need no parachutes, hairs or wings to help them fly. Airplanes have been used to collect grass seeds 3,000 feet in the air! Orchid seeds are as fine as dust. Just one ripe orchid pod holds millions. If you breathe on them gently, they billow up like a cloud. The wind can blow tiny seeds like these for a few hundred miles.

Other seeds use the wind to travel along the ground. Some seeds fall after the first snow, and the wind sends them sledding over the frozen surface. When the snow melts, they may sink down to the earth and start to grow.

Other seeds cartwheel across the ground. Have you ever seen big, brown tumbleweeds blowing across a desert or prairie? When these bushes are full of ripe seeds, they dry out and the roots shrivel up. Then the first wind to come along uproots the plant and rolls it along the ground, scattering seeds as it goes.

Can you imagine plants that snap, crackle and pop? Tap the touch-me-not's seed pod and it explodes with a *snap!* The pod is made of five little strips that grow tighter and tighter over the seeds inside. When ripe, the strips spring apart at the slightest touch. They hit the seeds and flip them in all directions. The seed pod of the wild geranium is spring-loaded, too. But its seeds are attached to the springs. When the springs snap, they throw out the seeds the way you throw a baseball.

Have you ever pinched a slippery watermelon seed between your thumb and finger and popped it away? This is how violet and witch hazel plants scatter their seeds. The sides of the seed pods open at one end and squeeze harder and harder on the seeds inside. Pinch, POP!

Some seeds hitchhike. The next time your dog bites at a sticker in his fur, look for the hooks or claws the seed uses to hitch a ride. Cockleburs, burdocks and sticktights all travel like this. They are bitten, brushed or bumped off somewhere along the way to begin another pesky plant.

You help seeds travel, too, when you pop a touch-me-not pod or when cockleburs stick to your socks. And where did you toss last summer's watermelon seeds?

1. This passage tells us
   - ☐ a. why plants produce seeds.
   - ☐ b. how seeds scatter.
   - ☐ c. about edible seeds.
   - ☐ d. what seeds need in order to grow.

2. Choose the main idea.
   - ☐ a. Many seeds have different ways of traveling.
   - ☐ b. Not every seed will sprout.
   - ☐ c. Most seeds can be used in the kitchen.
   - ☐ d. A fully ripe seed is useless.

3. Grass seeds have been found
   - ☐ a. 300 feet below the earth's surface.
   - ☐ b. frozen in the Arctic wastelands.
   - ☐ c. on the ocean floor.
   - ☐ d. 3,000 feet in the air.

4. In order to sprout, seeds usually
   - ☐ a. move away from the parent plant.
   - ☐ b. have to be big and heavy.
   - ☐ c. need to be fertilized.
   - ☐ d. become very cold and eventually pop.

5. Maple, elm and pine seeds can be compared to helicopters because
   - ☐ a. they do not glide when they fly.
   - ☐ b. they can't stay in the air very long.
   - ☐ c. they don't have parachutes.
   - ☐ d. they have wings that whirl.

6. A good synonym for shrivel is
   - ☐ a. uproot.
   - ☐ b. shrink.
   - ☐ c. pop.
   - ☐ d. swell.

CATEGORIES OF COMPREHENSION QUESTIONS

No. 1: Subject Matter	No. 3: Supporting Details	No. 5: Clarifying Devices
No. 2: Main Idea	No. 4: Conclusion	No. 6: Vocabulary in Context

19. THE UNDERWATER TIGER

Down in the dark waters of a pond lurks a fierce creature that is terribly ugly! Yet, scientists call it a *nymph*, a name given long ago to very beautiful maidens of the sea.

This water nymph starts life as an egg. It is usually attached to the stem of a water plant near the pond's surface. When the creature breaks out of the egg in the springtime, it is small and soft.

Suddenly, the stems of the water plants quiver, and the nymph sees something flash like silver. Quickly it lets its body drop softly down into the mud. It does not know that the silvery flash was made by a fish, but it does know that such a strange movement may mean a big mouth is near to gobble it up.

So, the water nymph hides in the muck and soon grows a hard body covering. This hard shell is actually the water nymph's outer skeleton. If you looked closely at this creature, you would also see that it now has six powerful legs, the legs of an insect.

What an ugly, dangerous-looking creature it soon becomes! It seems to grow in sudden spurts instead of gradually. For a while, it slowly wanders around feeding on smaller creatures but staying exactly the same size. Then one day it goes into hiding. The inner body, which day by day had grown too big, suddenly forces the outer skeleton to split. Out of this climbs the soft body inside. It is so soft at first that it must stay hidden until it can grow new armor. When it finally emerges, it is a bigger nymph. It continues to grow bigger and bigger by these strange leaps and bounds. Every two weeks or so it again goes into hiding, splits and casts off its outer shell, and soon emerges as a larger nymph. It will repeat this process about nine times during its life.

Now at last it is a true water nymph, so fierce looking that it has few enemies. Since it is a kind of mud-brown color, it is not easy to see on the muddy bottom. Its color hides it not only from enemies but also from those insects and tiny fish it wants to catch and eat.

When the water nymph gets as big and ugly as it is ever going to, it moves about restlessly on the bottom and looks up eagerly toward the light. At last it sluggishly climbs a water-plant stem. Up and up it goes until it breaks through the water into the air and sunlight. When its body is dry, its armor-like skeleton breaks open for the last time. But this time, no ugly water nymph comes out.

Out comes a king of the air indeed! Its great clear wings slowly unfold. The soft body begins to harden and glisten in the sunshine. The ugly water nymph has at long last become a lovely dragonfly.

1. This story is about the
   ☐ a. growth of a dragonfly.
   ☐ b. dragonfly's dinner.
   ☐ c. death of a dragonfly.
   ☐ d. female dragonfly.

2. A nymph is
   ☐ a. a female dragonfly.
   ☐ b. a dragonfly egg.
   ☐ c. the dragonfly's wings.
   ☐ d. a young dragonfly.

3. Before reaching adulthood, the dragonfly will split its outer skeleton about
   ☐ a. three times.
   ☐ b. nine times.
   ☐ c. twelve times.
   ☐ d. fifteen times.

4. Dragonflies live in and near
   ☐ a. fresh water.
   ☐ b. coal mines.
   ☐ c. salt water.
   ☐ d. quicksand.

5. In the third paragraph the nymph was frightened by a
   ☐ a. sudden wind.
   ☐ b. bolt of lightning.
   ☐ c. loud noise.
   ☐ d. shiny object.

6. When a plant quivers, it
   ☐ a. dies.
   ☐ b. sheds its leaves.
   ☐ c. grows.
   ☐ d. shakes.

CATEGORIES OF COMPREHENSION QUESTIONS

No. 1: Subject Matter   No. 3: Supporting Details   No. 5: Clarifying Devices
No. 2: Main Idea   No. 4: Conclusion   No. 6: Vocabulary in Context

20. ANTS ON THE MOVE

Most ants can find their way across a large stretch of sand where there are no <u>landmarks</u>. Their secret is the sun! The ants also use the sun as an ever-present guidepost in finding their way back to the nest.

You and I know that the position of the sun in the sky changes all through the day. This means that even though the ant lines up with the sun, the sun's position will change while the ant is out looking for food. Doesn't this confuse the ant and cause it to lose its way? It doesn't because the ant has an internal clock which takes care of the sun's movement. When it leaves the nest, an ant somehow notices the position of the sun. By "remembering" this, the ant can find its way back home.

Do ants lose their way if the sun is hiding behind clouds? The answer is "no" — the ants still find their way back home. They have unusual eyes that can tell exactly where the sun is in the sky. This is because their eyes can see "polarized" light. This is a kind of light that comes from the sun even if the sky is cloudy. Ants can see what direction this light is coming from and so always know the position of the sun.

There is still another method that ants use to find their way around called "trail-making." This is especially important because it is the main way ants get their food.

When an ant is alone and finds food, it has a way to let the ants back at the nest know where the food is. It does this by "making a trail." On its trip from the food supply back to the nest, the ant leaves a liquid on the ground. This liquid has a special smell. When the ant arrives at the nest, it does not even have to meet another ant — the odor from the trail is enough to lead them. The others then follow the trail smell right to the food. Then they all work to carry the food back to the nest.

If you ever see a long line of ants marching back and forth along the same narrow path, you can be sure that they are following the smell of the trail. But ants do not have noses, so how can they smell the trail?

Ants smell with their antennae. These are the two hairlike projections that jut out from the tops of the ants' heads. On each antenna there are over 1,000 smaller hairs that serve as smellers and feelers. If you watch an ant very closely, you will see that its antennae are always moving. This constant motion shows that the insect is always smelling and feeling what is around it.

1. This story tells how ants
   ☐ a. make their tunnels.
   ☐ b. and aphids live together.
   ☐ c. find their way.
   ☐ d. care for their young.

2. According to this article, ants
   ☐ a. use the sun and trail-making to guide them.
   ☐ b. eat the sweet tasting liquid given off by the aphids.
   ☐ c. do not survive very long in an ant farm.
   ☐ d. live a long active life.

3. Ants smell with their
   ☐ a. tongues.
   ☐ b. antennae.
   ☐ c. teeth.
   ☐ d. abdomen.

4. Which of the following is most likely true?
   ☐ a. Ants live together in groups.
   ☐ b. Not all ants survive the cold winter.
   ☐ c. Ants are only found in certain parts of the world.
   ☐ d. Young ants care for themselves.

5. If the sun is hiding behind clouds, the day could be described as
   ☐ a. sunshiny and cheerful.
   ☐ b. windy and bright.
   ☐ c. dark and cloudy.
   ☐ d. sunny and warm.

6. A landmark is used
   ☐ a. to fool the ant.
   ☐ b. to hide the ant.
   ☐ c. to destroy the ant.
   ☐ d. to guide the ant.

CATEGORIES OF COMPREHENSION QUESTIONS

No. 1: Subject Matter   No. 3: Supporting Details   No. 5: Clarifying Devices
No. 2: Main Idea   No. 4: Conclusion   No. 6: Vocabulary in Context

21. THE HAYMAKER

The haymaker is really a pika. It is small and gray and is the softest furry animal I know. Only 6 to 8 inches long, it weighs only about 6 ounces when fully grown.

Pikas are found only in the western United States. They live high in the mountains among jumbled masses of fallen rock known as talus (TAY luss). Some kinds of ground squirrels also live in such places. They pass the winter in the deep sleep of hibernation, but the pika does not. Like members of the rabbit family, pikas are active all year round.

The pika prepares for winter during warm summer days. Like a farmer, it makes hay while the sun shines. The pika cuts grass and spreads it out on the rocks to dry. If a sudden shower comes up, the pika dashes out and brings the grass under cover. When the storm passes the pika again spreads the grass out to dry.

Hay is stored somewhere under the rocks or in cracks where it cannot get wet. The snow that blankets the mountains keeps everything beneath it warmer than the outside air. Here the pika lives protected from the bitter cold. The pika's store of hay keeps it well fed throughout the long months of winter. Each little pika will store many armfuls of hay. In the olden days, if the Shoshoni Indians found hay under the rocks, they took it to feed their horses.

Pikas are noisy little creatures. You could probably hear their whistling chirp before you could actually see one. Pikas are most active early in the morning or late in the evening. The soles of their feet are padded, and they have sharp toenails which help them get a good grip on the rocks upon which they climb. The pikas usually live in small colonies. They run among the rocks and, because they are so small, it is really hard to get a good look at them.

Pikas certainly make some of the bleak mountaintops a lot livelier. If you should go on a vacation trip to some of the western mountains, keep alert and watch for them. When you come back home, you can tell your friends, "I saw one of America's least known animals." They probably won't even know about the pika.

1. The haymaker spends the winter in the same way that
   ☐ a. rabbits do.
   ☐ b. ground squirrels do.
   ☐ c. bears do.
   ☐ d. geese do.

2. Pikas live
   ☐ a. on the wide prairies.
   ☐ b. in low-lying swamp areas.
   ☐ c. in the western mountain areas of the U.S.
   ☐ d. only in the southern states.

3. The skin of the pika is
   ☐ a. feathery.
   ☐ b. scaly.
   ☐ c. fleshy.
   ☐ d. furry.

4. The pika gets ready for the long winter months by
   ☐ a. storing food.
   ☐ b. moving its burrow.
   ☐ c. migrating.
   ☐ d. growing a thicker skin.

5. Pikas can be described as
   ☐ a. lazy.
   ☐ b. quiet.
   ☐ c. mean.
   ☐ d. lively.

6. Bleak mountaintops are
   ☐ a. colorful.
   ☐ b. tree covered.
   ☐ c. bare.
   ☐ d. grassy.

CATEGORIES OF COMPREHENSION QUESTIONS

No. 1: Subject Matter No. 3: Supporting Details No. 5: Clarifying Devices
No. 2: Main Idea No. 4: Conclusion No. 6: Vocabulary in Context

22. OUR GRASSLANDS

One hundred and fifty years ago great numbers of bison, pronghorn, turkeys, quail and other animals and birds roamed the North American prairies. They ate the wild grasses that covered millions of acres with a thick, tough sod.

As white settlers moved west, they brought herds of cattle and sheep. These grass eaters also fed on the ranges. Soon there was not enough food for them and for the wild animals as well.

Pioneers killed the wild animals for meat and skins, leaving the grass for livestock. Huge cattle herds ate more and more of the grass. As they were driven to market, they trampled and damaged the grasslands.

In 1881 Congress passed the Homestead Act, giving 160 acres of land to anyone who would live on it, plow it and plant crops. Homesteaders plowed the sod, destroying more of the grasslands, and planted wheat and other grains.

These new crops grew well in many places, but sometimes there was not enough water for grain. The sod that had soaked up rain like a sponge and had held the water was now gone. Topsoil washed away in gullies, and blew away with the prairie winds

Finally, people understood the importance of the grasslands. They knew that they must do something to stop the destruction of it. During the past fifty years, a science called "range management" has helped save and improve natural pastures.

Excellent natural grasslands are increasing in the United States. Many plowed fields have returned to grass. Grass is the best crop for restoring land that has been worn out by other crops or by overgrazing.

Grass is also the cheapest known food for cattle and sheep and one of the best. But care is now taken to limit the number of cattle or sheep which graze on a certain area. Enough of each grass plant is left after grazing to grow and make seeds for a new crop.

1. This passage is mainly about North America's
   - ☐ a. wetlands.
   - ☐ b. forests.
   - ☐ c. prairies.
   - ☐ d. deserts.

2. The writer is explaining
   - ☐ a. why range wars happened.
   - ☐ b. how the destruction of the grassland came about.
   - ☐ c. how to find good topsoil.
   - ☐ d. why the bison suddenly disappeared.

3. In 1881 Congress passed the
   - ☐ a. Intolerable Acts.
   - ☐ b. Homestead Act.
   - ☐ c. Monroe Doctrine.
   - ☐ d. Civil Rights Act.

4. The grasslands
   - ☐ a. were wastelands.
   - ☐ b. supported very little life.
   - ☐ c. held the soil together.
   - ☐ d. are dry and hot.

5. The writer feels that the grasslands should be
   - ☐ a. eliminated.
   - ☐ b. flooded.
   - ☐ c. replaced.
   - ☐ d. protected.

6. Another word for <u>sod</u> is
   - ☐ a. meat.
   - ☐ b. underbrush.
   - ☐ c. turf.
   - ☐ d. gullies.

CATEGORIES OF COMPREHENSION QUESTIONS

No. 1: Subject Matter	No. 3: Supporting Details	No. 5: Clarifying Devices
No. 2: Main Idea	No. 4: Conclusion	No. 6: Vocabulary in Context

23. UTTERLY RIDICULOUS

When men exploring Australia discovered the platypus in the early 1800s, they sent skins and descriptions of the funny animal back to Europe. Animal experts from many nations saw this strange new animal and began to quarrel about it. "An animal with fur and webbed feet and a bill like a duck's! Impossible!" some said. "A mammal which lays eggs! Ridiculous!" said others.

These educated men just couldn't believe such an animal really existed. It couldn't be a reptile because it was warm-blooded. It couldn't be a mammal because it laid eggs. It couldn't be a bird because it had no wings or feathers. Some even said they were being tricked — that the platypus didn't exist at all. But they were wrong. The platypus lived then, and he lives today to amaze us all. He is one of two known mammals in the whole world which breed their young by laying eggs!

This furry little animal is about 20 inches long. His tail is long and flat, something like a beaver's. He has a broad, flat bill like a duck's — in fact, the platypus is called a "duckbill."

Another interesting thing about this shy, little fellow is that he spends a lot of his time in the water as well as on land. He is *semiaquatic*. Morning and evening he goes into the water to find his food on the bottoms of streams. He may dive underwater and stay under for as long as five minutes while searching for worms, the eggs of water insects, tiny shelled animals and small fish. Although the platypus has keen eyesight and hearing on land, he is completely blind and deaf underwater because he covers his eyes and ears with folds of skin to keep the water out. Only a highly developed sense of touch in his bill guides him to food.

Now, don't you agree that the platypus must have been very confusing to the men who first discovered him? But wait. This fascinating little creature has more surprises in store for you. When he is in the water, he has webbed feet like a duck's to help him swim. When he returns to dry land, he folds back the webs to uncover claws on his front feet. These claws help him walk and dig his burrows!

Even today, mystery surrounds the amazing platypus despite all that modern science has learned about him. The male platypus, for example, has two poison-filled spurs on his rear legs, but no one knows why. Some people think he uses them to kill his <u>rivals</u> in the lovers' duel for a mate, but that is just a guess.

1. The platypus is
   ☐ a. a mammal.
   ☐ b. a reptile.
   ☐ c. a bird.
   ☐ d. an amphibian.

2. The main idea of this passage is that the platypus is
   ☐ a. rapidly dying out.
   ☐ b. dangerous.
   ☐ c. unusual.
   ☐ d. a common bird.

3. The platypus was discovered in the
   ☐ a. early 1800s.
   ☐ b. middle 1800s.
   ☐ c. late 1800s.
   ☐ d. early 1900s.

4. This article leads us to believe that most mammals
   ☐ a. live in the water.
   ☐ b. have fur.
   ☐ c. are cold blooded.
   ☐ d. do not lay eggs.

5. How did some early scientists first feel about the platypus?
   ☐ a. They were afraid of it.
   ☐ b. They were bored with it.
   ☐ c. They were sure it did not exist.
   ☐ d. They disliked it.

6. As used in this passage, a <u>rival</u> is
   ☐ a. a neighbor.
   ☐ b. an enemy.
   ☐ c. a mate.
   ☐ d. a friend.

CATEGORIES OF COMPREHENSION QUESTIONS

No. 1: Subject Matter   No. 3: Supporting Details   No. 5: Clarifying Devices
No. 2: Main Idea   No. 4: Conclusion   No. 6: Vocabulary in Context

24. A GIANT IN DANGER

Would you save a giant's life? A wonderful old giant? Of course you would, if you could! Well, there *is* a giant whose life is in danger, and you can help him. His name is Saguaro (su WAH ro). If you have not seen Saguaro in his home in Arizona, I'll bet you have seen him many times on TV or in movies about the West. "He" is a big cactus plant that stands like a giant with armlike branches raised.

What a fascinating plant the saguaro is! It starts life as a tiny seed not much bigger than a large grain of sand. It is one of nearly 2,000 seeds that develop at the same time within a single flower.

If a saguaro seed sprouts on bare ground, it usually dies in the hot desert sun. But a seed that falls among thick bushes and weeds is shaded and usually survives. Also, the new plant that sprouts from it is hidden from the rodents which eat small saguaros.

In its first season, a saguaro is only as big as a pea. After twenty-five years it is only 4 feet high. When it is 10 feet high, the saguaro is still a young giant, for then it is only from forty to fifty years old. It still has about a hundred years to live — if man or disease does not prevent its survival.

When it has been alive for about fifty years, there comes a May evening when something special happens to the saguaro. Beautiful white flowers appear on the tip ends of its branches. They will close by early afternoon of the next day, but before they do they provide sweet <u>nectar</u> for many insects and birds.

When the fruits ripen during June and July, the birds come back for another feast. As they have done for centuries, Pima and Papago Indians gather the fruits for food.

Saguaros grow in groups so large that they form a real forest. In this forest are gilded flickers and gila woodpeckers. Where do woodpeckers dig their nest holes? You guessed it — in the giant cactuses. When a hole is completed, the plant's sap hardens all around the inside of the hole. The plant is not harmed because nests are made during the season when the sap will harden quickly. Years later, after a cactus has fallen and rotted away, the tough, gourd-shaped nest linings can still be found in the remains. These are called "boots."

Each year the woodpeckers build new nests, so birds such as purple martins, sparrow hawks and elf owls move into the woodpeckers' old homes. Tap gently on the saguaro, and, if the owl is at home, its head will appear in the opening.

1. This article is about
   □ a. a plant.
   □ b. a mammal.
   □ c. an insect.
   □ d. a reptile.

2. According to this passage, the giant saguaro is
   □ a. very harmful.
   □ b. extinct.
   □ c. in danger.
   □ d. poisonous.

3. The saguaro lives
   □ a. in desert areas.
   □ b. on rocky cliffs.
   □ c. in the wetlands.
   □ d. underwater.

4. Parts of the saguaro are
   □ a. purple.
   □ b. filled with water.
   □ c. good to eat.
   □ d. sold for a high price.

5. When the writer states that during the "first season a saguaro is only as big as a pea," he is comparing
   □ a. shapes.   □ c. taste.
   □ b. colors.   □ d. sizes.

6. Nectar is the
   □ a. sap of a plant.
   □ b. sweet liquid of a plant.
   □ c. water used by a plant.
   □ d. minerals in a plant.

CATEGORIES OF COMPREHENSION QUESTIONS

No. 1: Subject Matter   No. 3: Supporting Details   No. 5: Clarifying Devices
No. 2: Main Idea   No. 4: Conclusion   No. 6: Vocabulary in Context

---

25. SAVE THE GIANT

The white-winged dove visits the saguaro forests where it feeds on the flowers and fruit. In so doing it covers its face and body with the yellow pollen. Then the pollen gets spread from one blossom to another, helping to pollinate the cactuses.

The saguaro's life is threatened mostly by two enemies — man and disease. Even though it is a 30-foot giant weighing 10 tons, man can kill it in an instant. But why would anyone want to kill such a handsome plant? Unfortunately, persons we call vandals think it is fun to destroy things. They drive up to a saguaro cactus and push it over with their automobile bumper. In one second they destroy a desert giant that has lived in peace for perhaps 150 years or more. Other vandals "stab" saguaros by throwing sharp stones at them just to see the stones stick in the fleshy covering. This weakens the plants and allows bacteria to enter. Some persons prefer to shoot holes in the giant plants, but the effects are the same. The saguaro is doomed when any of these things is done to it.

Have you heard stories about how men dying of thirst have gotten water from the saguaro as they might from a big jug? The stories are not true. Saguaros do store water, but there is no juglike cavity inside the plant. Its liquid is held in the same way as the juice inside a melon. But saguaro juice is like glue and has a bad taste. It will irritate your throat and actually make you more thirsty. By storing tons of water in its own body, a saguaro can live for two years without rain. When a drought lasts a long time, though, weak and diseased cactuses often die.

Just the same, some persons are not satisfied until they have cut down a saguaro and found this out for themselves. Others chop down the plants just to see what they look like inside.

The saguaro has natural enemies, too. A little moth carries bacteria from one saguaro to another and this kills some of the cactuses. Rodents, moths and the hot sun destroy many young saguaros. These are nature's ways of keeping saguaros from becoming too numerous.

Saguaros have been successful in surviving for millions of years, far longer than man has lived on earth. Let's not be among those who destroy this giant of plants.

1. This article is about a giant
   ☐ a. tree.
   ☐ b. whale.
   ☐ c. cactus.
   ☐ d. squid.

2. The two most important enemies of the saguaro are
   ☐ a. man and disease.
   ☐ b. raging rivers and ice.
   ☐ c. pollution and rain.
   ☐ d. smoke and oil slicks.

3. The giant saguaro may weigh as much as
   ☐ a. 2 tons.
   ☐ b. 4 tons.
   ☐ c. 7 tons.
   ☐ d. 10 tons.

4. Which of the following is most likely true?
   ☐ a. The saguaro can store water for long periods of time.
   ☐ b. Saguaros are becoming too numerous.
   ☐ c. Saguaro juice is very tasty.
   ☐ d. Many stories have been written about the saguaro's life.

5. The juice of the saguaro is like glue. This means it is
   ☐ a. harmful.
   ☐ b. good to eat.
   ☐ c. sticky.
   ☐ d. hot.

6. As used in this article, a cavity is
   ☐ a. a small scratch.
   ☐ b. harmful germs.
   ☐ c. fleshy skin.
   ☐ d. a hollow space.

CATEGORIES OF COMPREHENSION QUESTIONS

No. 1: Subject Matter	No. 3: Supporting Details	No. 5: Clarifying Devices
No. 2: Main Idea	No. 4: Conclusion	No. 6: Vocabulary in Context

ACKNOWLEDGEMENTS

The articles appearing in this booklet have been reprinted with the kind permission of the following publications and publishers to whom the author is indebted:

Aramco World Magazine, published by The Arabian American Oil Company, New York, New York.

The Communicator, published by the New York State Outdoor Education Association, Syracuse, New York.

The Conservationist, published by the New York State Conservation Department, Albany, New York.

A Cornell Science Leaflet, published by the New York State College of Agriculture and Life Sciences, a unit of the State University, at Cornell University, Ithaca, New York.

Food, The Yearbook of Agriculture, published by the United States Department of Agriculture, Washington, D.C.

Handbook of Nature-Study, published by Comstock Publishing Company, Ithaca, New York.

Kansas Fish & Game, published by the Kansas Forestry, Fish and Game Commission, Pratt, Kansas.

National Wildlife, published by The National Wildlife Federation, Washington, D.C.

Outdoor Oklahoma, published by the Oklahoma Department of Wildlife Conservation, Oklahoma City, Oklahoma.

Pennsylvania Game News, published by the Pennsylvania Game Commission, Harrisburg, Pennsylvania.

Ranger Rick's Nature Magazine, published by The National Wildlife Federation, Washington, D.C.

The Tennessee Conservationist, published by the Tennessee Department of Conservation and the Tennessee Game and Fish Commission.

ANSWER KEY

Passage 1:	1-b	2-d	3-a	4-b	5-d	6-b
Passage 2:	1-b	2-a	3-b	4-c	5-d	6-c
Passage 3:	1-d	2-a	3-b	4-c	5-d	6-a
Passage 4:	1-c	2-d	3-a	4-c	5-c	6-d
Passage 5:	1-a	2-d	3-b	4-b	5-c	6-b
Passage 6:	1-c	2-a	3-b	4-d	5-a	6-c
Passage 7:	1-a	2-b	3-d	4-a	5-c	6-c
Passage 8:	1-c	2-d	3-a	4-d	5-c	6-d
Passage 9:	1-d	2-c	3-b	4-b	5-d	6-a
Passage 10:	1-b	2-a	3-d	4-c	5-b	6-d
Passage 11:	1-b	2-d	3-d	4-b	5-c	6-d
Passage 12:	1-a	2-d	3-c	4-a	5-c	6-d
Passage 13:	1-a	2-c	3-b	4-d	5-d	6-b
Passage 14:	1-a	2-c	3-d	4-b	5-d	6-c
Passage 15:	1-a	2-b	3-d	4-a	5-b	6-b
Passage 16:	1-b	2-d	3-a	4-a	5-a	6-c
Passage 17:	1-c	2-d	3-a	4-b	5-a	6-d
Passage 18:	1-b	2-a	3-d	4-a	5-d	6-b
Passage 19:	1-a	2-d	3-b	4-a	5-d	6-d
Passage 20:	1-c	2-a	3-b	4-a	5-c	6-d
Passage 21:	1-a	2-c	3-d	4-a	5-d	6-c
Passage 22:	1-c	2-b	3-b	4-c	5-d	6-c
Passage 23:	1-a	2-c	3-a	4-d	5-c	6-b
Passage 24:	1-a	2-c	3-a	4-c	5-d	6-b
Passage 25:	1-c	2-a	3-d	4-a	5-c	6-d

DIAGNOSTIC CHART

READING PASSAGE::	1	2	3	4	5	6	7	8	9	10	11	12	13	14	15	16	17	18	19	20	21	22	23	24	25
1. SUBJECT MATTER																									
2. MAIN IDEAS																									
3. SUPPORTING DETAILS																									
4. CONCLUSIONS																									
5. CLARIFYING DEVICES																									
6. VOCABULARY																									

CATEGORIES OF COMPREHENSION SKILLS

GRAPHING YOUR PROGRESS

	1	2	3	4	5	6	7	8	9	10	11	12	13	14	15	16	17	18	19	20	21	22	23	24	25
6 CORRECT = 100%																									
5 CORRECT = 83%																									
4 CORRECT = 67%																									
3 CORRECT = 50%																									
2 CORRECT = 33%																									
1 CORRECT = 17%																									